HOW MANY SETS AND REPS SHOULD I DO

SIMPLE GUIDE TO EXERCISE

A.D RAMS

Contents

CHAPTER ONE

INTRODUCTION

Finding the ideal quantity of sets and repetitions for your exercise regimen is crucial to successfully reaching your fitness objectives. Understanding how many sets and reps to execute will help you customize your exercises to maximize results while avoiding the danger of injury or burnout, whether your goals are to gain muscle, enhance strength, or boost endurance. In this article, we'll go over the things to think about when figuring out how many sets and repetitions are right for your own needs and goals. We'll also offer suggestions for various fitness goals.

Understanding sets and reps is crucial while doing strength training

Gaining the best possible results from strength training and moving forward in your fitness path requires an understanding of sets and reps. This is the reason it matters:

Muscle Adaptation: The volume and intensity of your exercises, which are vital in promoting muscle growth and adaptation, are determined by the number of sets and repetitions. You may efficiently target particular muscle groups and provide the required stimulation for muscle growth and strength increases by knowing how many sets and reps to execute.

Progressive stress: You may gradually stress your muscles over time with proper set and rep manipulation, which is crucial for ongoing gains in strength and muscular mass. Through incremental increases in resistance, volume, or intensity, you can put your muscles through a struggle that will eventually cause them to adapt and strengthen.

Training Efficiency: By ensuring that you're working out successfully without overtraining or undertraining, knowing the right amount of sets and reps helps you maximize your training efficiency. You can make the most of your gym time and get greater results faster by planning your exercises with the ideal ratio of volume to intensity.

Injury Prevention: Having a solid understanding of sets and reps enables you to create well-rounded training plans that include an emphasis on technique, form, and recuperation. You may lower your chance of overuse injuries and make sure your muscles have enough time to rest and recover between exercises by avoiding excessive volume or intensity.

Goal Specificity: Whether you want to increase muscle mass, strength, endurance, or general fitness, you may customize sets and repetitions to meet your unique fitness objectives. You can optimize your exercises for the intended result by changing your training parameters to match your goals.

All things considered, mastering sets and reps in strength training gives you the ability to create efficient exercise plans that increase muscle mass, strength, and general fitness while lowering the chance of burnout or injury. You may advance your training and get the outcomes you want by learning how to adjust these factors according to your unique requirements and objectives.

Recognizing Sets and Reps

Achieving fitness objectives and creating efficient workout regimens require a fundamental understanding of sets and reps. Here's an explanation of sets and repetitions and how they benefit your training:

Sets: A set is a collection of consecutive, rest-free repetitions of an exercise. For instance, you have finished one set of push-ups if you accomplish ten push-ups in a succession without stopping for a rest. Sets are a useful tool for planning your workout and determining how much work is required for each exercise.

Repetitions (Reps): The amount of times you complete a certain exercise or movement in a single set is known as a repetition, or rep. For example, you have completed 10 repetitions of push-ups if you can accomplish 10 push-ups in a succession without pausing. The number of repetitions determines each set's workload and intensity.

Workout volume is the overall amount of work done during a training session. It is commonly expressed as the total number of sets, repetitions, and weight lifted. When it comes to promoting strength and muscle growth, volume is essential.

The degree of effort or resistance used during exercise is referred to as intensity, and it is frequently influenced by variables including the weight lifted, the speed at which the activity is performed, and the rest intervals in between sets. Greater resistance or heavier weights are usually used in higher intensity workouts, which can result in larger strength increases.

Progressive Overload: To encourage muscular growth and adaptation, progressive overload involves progressively raising the demands made on your muscles over time. To consistently test your muscles, you can accomplish this by gradually increasing the amount of sets, repetitions, or weight lifted during your workouts.

Muscle Hypertrophy: To achieve muscle hypertrophy, or muscle growth, it is usually advised to perform a moderate number of sets and reps with a moderate to heavy weight. For each exercise, this usually entails completing 3–4 sets of 8–12 repetitions, using a weight that will cause muscular fatigue at the end of each set.

Strength Development: Lower rep ranges with heavier weights are usually utilized to concentrate on building strength. This could entail utilizing a weight that is difficult but still permits you to retain correct form and technique for three to five sets of four to six repetitions per exercise.

Endurance Training: Higher repetition ranges with lesser weights are frequently used to increase muscle endurance. This could entail utilizing a weight that enables you to achieve the appropriate number of repetitions with proper form while completing 2-3 sets of 12–20 reps for each exercise.

Gaining control over sets and repetitions enables you to customize your training to meet your individual objectives, be they boosting strength, building muscle, increasing endurance, or improving general fitness. You can create training regimens that support your fitness goals and provide significant benefits by modifying these factors according to your unique demands and progress.

Variables Affecting Set and Rep Schemas

A workout program's choice of set and rep patterns is influenced by a number of factors. Having a thorough understanding of these elements is essential to creating a customized and successful training program. Here are some important things to think about:

Fitness Goals: Choosing the right set and rep schemes for your workouts is heavily influenced by your fitness goals. For instance, you can choose to use moderate weights and greater rep ranges (8–12 reps each set) if your objective is to gain muscle mass (hypertrophy). Lower rep ranges (1-6 reps each set) with heavier weights are usually employed if your objective is to improve strength.

Training Experience: The set and rep schemes that work best for you depend on your degree of training experience. As they develop strength and skill in their lifting techniques, beginners might find it beneficial to begin with higher rep ranges and work their way down to heavier weights and lower rep ranges.

Muscle Fiber Composition: Type I and Type II muscle fibers, which have different amounts of slow and fast twitch, are found in different muscle groups. Training adaptations can be maximized by designing sets and rep schemes that specifically target particular muscle fiber types. For instance, higher rep ranges target slow-twitch muscle fibers, which contribute to endurance, whereas lower rep ranges with heavier weights predominantly target fast-twitch muscle fibers, which are responsible for strength and power.

Training Intensity: The amount of resistance or effort used during an exercise is referred to as training intensity. Higher resistance or heavier weights are usually used in higher-intensity workouts, and shorter rep ranges may be necessary to handle the increased load. In contrast, higher rep ranges with smaller weights may be used in lower-intensity exercises to develop muscle endurance or metabolic conditioning.

Volume and Frequency: The choice of set and rep schemes is also influenced by the overall volume (sets x reps x weight) and frequency (number of workouts per week) of your training program. While lower-volume training plans might emphasize using heavier weights and shorter rep ranges to maximize strength gains, higher-volume training plans might include moderate to high rep ranges to build up enough workload for muscle growth.

Recovery Capacity: The amount and intensity of training you can handle depends on how well you recuperate from sessions.

CHAPTER TWO

Higher recovery capacities may enable people to tolerate higher training volumes and frequencies, which would enable them to perform more sets and repetitions throughout a workout. On the other hand, lower volume, higher intensity workouts may be beneficial for individuals with worse recovery capacities in order to avoid overtraining and encourage sufficient recovery.

Individual Preferences: When choosing set and rep schemes, personal preferences including exercise enjoyment, training style, and adherence to particular rep ranges should also be taken into account. While some people might love the burn and pump of higher repetitions at lower weights, others could like the challenge of heavier lifting at lower rep ranges.

Through careful consideration of these variables and customization of set and rep schemes to your unique objectives, degree of experience, and personal traits, you can create a comprehensive and efficient exercise regimen that optimizes your training results and fosters sustained advancements in strength, muscle mass, endurance, or general fitness.

Calculating Repetition Distances

The right range of repetitions for each set and rep depends on a number of variables, such as your personal preferences, training history, and fitness objectives. Here's how to figure out what your workouts' ideal repetition ranges are:

Establish Your Fitness Objectives: To begin, make sure your objectives are well-defined. Your goals will determine the ideal repetition ranges to reach your objectives, whether they be to develop muscle mass, strength, muscular endurance, or general fitness.

Think About Your Training Experience: Choosing the right repetition ranges requires careful consideration of your training background. Higher repetition ranges are a good place for beginners to start in order to build work capacity, optimal technique, and muscle endurance. You can gradually reduce the repetition ranges to concentrate on strength and hypertrophy as you get stronger and more experienced.

Recognize the Repetition Ranges:

Strength (1-6 reps): To achieve maximum strength, lower repetition ranges using heavier weights are usually utilized. Use a weight that permits you to attain muscular failure within the intended rep range and perform 1-6 reps each set.

Hypertrophy (6–12 reps): For muscle hypertrophy (growth), moderate repetition ranges are frequently utilized. Use a weight that makes you tired at the end of each set and aim for 6–12 repetitions per set.

Endurance (12+ reps): To increase muscle endurance and metabolic fitness, higher repetition ranges are frequently used. Use a smaller weight and complete 12 or more repetitions per set to sustain muscle endurance for a longer amount of time.

Customize Repetition Ranges to Your Objectives:

Strength: To optimize strength improvements, focus on lower repetition ranges (1-6 repetitions) using heavier weights. Exercises that are considered compound include bench presses, overhead presses, deadlifts, and squats.

Hypertrophy: To promote muscular growth and hypertrophy, use intermediate repetition ranges (6–12 reps). A range of isolation and compound workouts can be employed to focus on distinct muscle groups.

Endurance: To increase muscular endurance and cardiovascular conditioning, focus on higher repetition ranges (12+ repetitions) with smaller weights. Your routines should incorporate bodyweight exercises, circuit training, and high-rep sets.

Periodize Your Training: If possible, divide your program into phases that are concentrated on various repetition ranges. For example, to target different components of fitness and avoid plateaus, you could alternate between phases of strength, hypertrophy, and endurance training.

Listen to Your Body: Modify your training based on your observations of how your body reacts to varying repetition ranges. If you find it difficult to perform the required amount of reps with good technique every time, think about varying the weight or range of repetitions to make sure you're safe and getting the intended results.

Progress Over Time: Gradually strain your muscles to push yourself beyond your comfort zone. To encourage continuous improvement and adaptability, progressively increase the weight lifted, the number of sets, or the intensity of your exercises.

You can maximize your workouts and reach your targeted fitness objectives by carefully evaluating your goals, experience level, and training preferences to identify the most optimal repetition ranges for your sets and reps. For long-term success, never forget to place a high priority on appropriate form, progression, and consistency in your training regimen.

Choosing Set Schemes

Choosing set schemes entails figuring out how many sets you'll do for every exercise in your training regimen. The following advice will assist you in selecting the best set schemes for your training objectives:

Think About Your Fitness Objectives:

Strength: Choose lower set patterns with heavier weights if your objective is to gain more strength. To concentrate on lifting hard and optimizing strength gains, aim for three to five sets per exercise.

Hypertrophy (Muscle Growth): Higher set plans are often advised in order to promote muscle growth. Use moderate weights for three to five sets per exercise to generate enough volume for muscular hypertrophy.

Endurance: Moderate to high set plans may be helpful when exercising for muscular endurance. To increase endurance, think about doing 2-4 sets of each exercise with lesser weights and higher repetition ranges.

Experience in Training:

Beginners: To enable adaptation and progressive advancement, beginners may begin with simpler set schemes. A foundation of strength and technique can be built by novices by beginning with two to three sets of each exercise.

Intermediate/Advanced: To keep pushing their muscles and encouraging growth, intermediate and advanced lifters could profit from higher set patterns. Try three to five sets of each exercise to get the best training stimulus.

Focus on Muscle Groups:

Compound Exercises: Higher set patterns help fully engage all muscle fibers during compound exercises that target several muscular groups, such as squats, deadlifts, and bench presses. For compound exercises, opt for three to five sets.

Exercises for Isolation: Less sets may be needed for exercises that concentrate on particular muscle regions (such as tricep extensions and bicep curls). For isolated exercises, aim for 2-4 sets in order to target and tire the muscles efficiently.

Volume and Recuperation:

Training Volume: To prevent overtraining and encourage proper recovery, balance the overall training volume with the set plans. Lower total volume per workout may be necessary for higher set schemes in order to avoid overexertion of fatigue.

Recovery: When choosing preset schemes, take your ability to recover into account. Choose lower set schemes if you're easily fatigued or have poor recovery capabilities in order to avoid overtraining and promote sufficient recuperation in between exercises.

Time Division:

Progressive Overload: To encourage progressive overload and avoid adaptation plateaus, periodize your training program by gradually modifying predetermined regimens. Use both higher and lower set scheme stages to mix up the training stimulus and keep improving.

Personal Preferences:

Training Enjoyment: When choosing set schemes, take your preferences and level of enjoyment from training into account. Higher intensity, lower set plans might be better if you like shorter, more intense workouts. greater set plans, on the other hand, can be more appropriate if you like longer, greater volume workouts.

Play around and Pay attention to your body:

Trial and error: Try out several regimens to see which one best suits your goals and physique. Track your development and modify the plans you've been given based on how each person responds to training.

Listen to Your Body: Observe how your body reacts to various regimens and make necessary adjustments. If you find yourself feeling overly tired, sore, or not making any progress, think about changing your set schemes to better fit your requirements.

You may create a comprehensive and successful exercise program that fits your fitness goals and encourages long-term success by taking these aspects into account and customizing your set schemes to your unique objectives, experience level, and tastes.

Recommendations for Various Training Objectives

For sets and repetitions suited to various training objectives, consider the following general guidelines:

Power

Sets: Try to complete 3-5 sets of each exercise.

Rep ranges 1-6 should be the main emphasis.

Intensity: Lift large weights until you are able to no longer perform the appropriate number of reps.

Rest: To ensure complete recovery, allow for lengthier rest intervals (2–5 minutes) in between sets.

Muscle growth, or hypertrophy:

Sets: Try to complete 3-5 sets of each exercise.

Rep ranges should be modest (6–12 reps).

Intensity: Use weights that permit good form even after each set, but that exhaust the user by the finish.

Rest: To maintain intensity, take shorter (60-90 seconds) rest intervals in between sets.

Physical stamina:

Add two to four sets to each exercise.

Reps: Concentrate on doing more repetitions (12+).

Intensity: Use lesser weights so that your form doesn't suffer and you can perform the necessary amount of repetitions.

Rest: To maintain cardiovascular demand, keep rest intervals brief (30–60 seconds).

Strength:

Sets: Use three to five sets for each exercise.

Reps: To emphasize explosive movements, use lower rep ranges (1–5).

Intensity: Quickly and maximally exert yourself while lifting moderate to heavy weights.

Rest: To sustain power production, give yourself enough time (2–5 minutes) in between sets.

Cardiovascular Endurance:

Sets: Add one to three sets to each workout or circuit.

Reps: Work out constantly for a predetermined amount of time (e.g., 30 seconds to 2 minutes).

Intensity: To raise heart rate, keep a constant tempo or up the intensity as necessary.

Rest: To maintain cardiovascular demand, take little time off in between workouts or circuits.

Practical Instruction:

Sets: Use two to four sets for each exercise or movement style.

Reps: To target different facets of functional fitness, use a range of rep ranges (e.g., 6–12 reps).

Intensity: Ensure that your workouts closely resemble the motions and obstacles you would face in real life.

Rest: Modify rest intervals in accordance with the particular requirements of every workout or circuit.

Keep in mind that these are only recommendations; each person's reaction to training will be different. It is critical to pay attention to your body, monitor your progress, and modify your sets and repetitions in accordance with your training history, goals, and preferences. Additionally, to avoid plateaus and modify sets, reps, and intensity over time, think about implementing periodization into your training routine. Speaking with a coach or fitness expert can also offer you individualized advice and assistance to help you successfully accomplish your training objectives.

Periodization and Difference

In order to maximize performance and avoid plateaus, periodization entails gradually changing training variables such as sets, reps, intensity, and volume. A crucial component of periodization is diversity in sets and reps, which enables focused response to various training stimuli. Periodization and variation in sets and reps can be included into a training program in the following ways:

Macrocycle:

Long-Term Planning: Break up your program into training modules, or macrocycles, which last anything from a few months to a year.

Phases: Include specific training phases, such as hypertrophy, strength, power, and peaking periods, inside each macrocycle.

Variation: Within each phase, modify the sets, repetitions, and intensity parameters to target particular adaptations and performance objectives.

Mesocycle:

Divide each macrocycle into mesocycles, which usually span a few weeks to a few months, for intermediate planning.

Focus Areas: Every mesocycle might concentrate on a different area of training, such as increasing power, endurance, or strength.

Progression: To encourage ongoing adaptation and advancement, progressively increase sets, repetitions, and intensity throughout each mesocycle.

Microcycle:

Short-Term Planning: Each mesocycle should be further divided into microcycles, each of which lasts for about a week.

Weekly Structure: Schedule your workouts with variations in sets, reps, exercises, and training modalities for every microcycle.

CHAPTER THREE

Periodization Models: Utilize various periodization models to adjust sets and reps within each microcycle, including block, undulating, and linear periodization.

Changes in Reps and Sets:

Strength Phase: To optimize neural adaptations and strength increases, concentrate on lower rep ranges (1-6 reps) with heavier weights during a strength phase.

Hypertrophy Phase: To promote muscular growth and hypertrophy, utilize moderate weights and moderate rep ranges (6–12 reps).

Endurance Phase: To increase muscle endurance and metabolic conditioning, employ higher rep ranges (12+ repetitions) with smaller weights during this phase.

Power Phase: To build speed, power, and athleticism, concentrate on lower rep ranges (1–5) using explosive motions and moderate–to–heavy weights.

Increasing Stress:

Gradual Progression: To encourage progressive overload and continuing adaptation, gradually increase the number of sets, repetitions, and/or intensity over time.

Periodic Deloads: To minimize the risk of overtraining, incorporate scheduled deload weeks or mesocycles to lower training volume and intensity. This will allow for recuperation and adaptation.

Customization:

Tailored Approach: When creating and executing periodized training programs, take into account individual aspects including training experience, capacity for recovery, goals, and preferences.

Adjustments: Based on individual answers and feedback, be ready to modify sets, reps, and other training factors.

You can methodically alter training stimuli to maximize performance, encourage ongoing improvement, and avoid training plateaus by including periodization and variation in sets and reps into your training program. Periodized training guarantees that your exercises stay tough, efficient, and long-lasting while enabling tailored adaptation to certain training goals.

Personal Aspects

It's important to take a few things into account when calculating sets and reps for a person's exercise program in order to customize the training schedule to meet their unique demands and objectives. The following are some particular things to think about:

Objectives for Fitness:

Recognize the person's main fitness objectives, whether they be to gain more muscle, become stronger, boost endurance, improve sports performance, or accomplish particular functional goals.

Choose sets and repetitions that correspond with their objectives; for example, use lower reps for maximal strength, moderate reps for hypertrophy, or greater reps for muscular endurance.

Experience in Training:

Consider the person's training background and knowledge with various workouts, training methods, and degrees of intensity.

Beginners can improve their form, neuromuscular coordination, and work capacity by beginning with easier exercises, lighter weights, and greater rep ranges.

For intermediate and advanced athletes to keep improving and avoid plateaus, they might need more intricate training regimens, greater weights, and different rep schemes.

Strengthening Degrees:

When recommending sets and repetitions, take into account the patient's present strength and lifting capabilities.

While people with lower strength levels may concentrate on developing a foundation of strength with lighter weights and greater rep ranges, those with higher strength levels may need to use heavier weights and shorter rep ranges to encourage additional strength improvements.

The composition of muscle fibers:

Understand that depending on genetics and training experience, different people may have varying amounts of fast-twitch versus slow-twitch muscle fiber types.

Adjust reps and sets to maximize training adaptations and focus on particular muscle fiber types. For instance, people who are more predisposed to fast-twitch fibers might benefit more from high-rep, high-intensity training, whereas others who are more predisposed to slow-twitch fibers might gain more from higher rep, lower-intensity training.

Past Injury History and Restrictions:

Think about any musculoskeletal restrictions, injuries from the past or present, or illnesses that could influence the type of exercise you choose and how hard you train.

Exercises that reduce the chance of exacerbating pre-existing injuries or conditions should be given priority. Adjust sets, reps, and sets as necessary to account for any physical restrictions or contraindications.

Recuperation Potential:

Evaluate the person's ability to recuperate, taking into account aspects including overall living habits, stress levels, food, and the quality of their sleep.

To avoid overtraining and maximize training adaptations, modify training volume, intensity, and frequency in accordance with their capacity to recuperate in between workouts.

Personal Preferences and Drive:

When creating an exercise regimen, take into account the person's training preferences, motivation, and style.

To improve adherence and long-term compliance with the program, include workouts, sets, and repetitions that suit their interests, training preferences, and level of enjoyment.

By keeping these specific factors in mind, you can create a tailored and successful training program that targets the particular requirements, objectives, and traits of every person, ultimately optimizing their chances of success and reaching the highest levels of fitness.

Advancement and Monitoring

Any great training program, including sets and reps, must include progression and tracking. Here's how to add these elements to your sets and reps routine:

Increasing Stress:

Increase the strain your muscles are under gradually over time to encourage ongoing adaptation and advancement.

Enhancing form and technique, adding sets or reps, lowering rest intervals between sets, and raising the weight lifted are all examples of progression.

Apply the idea of progressive overload in a methodical manner to guarantee steady improvements in strength, size of muscles, or endurance.

Gradual Rises:

Aim for gradual increases in volume or intensity while advancing sets and reps to prevent abrupt leaps that could cause overtraining or injury.

To give a progressive stimulus for adaptation and improvement, increase the number of sets, repetitions, or weight lifted by little increments (e.g., 5–10% every week).

Time Division:

To avoid adaptation plateaus and to alter sets, reps, and intensity over time, incorporate periodization into your training regimen.

To target distinct training goals, plan training phases with diverse emphasis (e.g., strength, hypertrophy, power) and modify sets and reps accordingly.

Monitoring Development:

Maintain thorough workout logs that include sets, reps, weights utilized, rest intervals, and perceived effort.

To measure your development over time and keep an eye on gains in strength, muscle size, endurance, or performance, use a training app, spreadsheet, or workout diary.

Examine and evaluate your training data on a regular basis to spot patterns, advantages, disadvantages, and areas that need work.

Benchmarks for Performance:

Determine precise performance standards or objectives for sets and reps according to your personal training goals and capacities.

Aim to increase performance indicators like total volume done, maximum weight lifted, and repetitions at a specific intensity gradually.

Self-Control:

Take note of how your body feels on any particular day and modify the number of sets and reps accordingly.

By modifying training volume and intensity in response to variables like tiredness, recovery state, stress levels, and general training preparation, you can practice auto-regulation.

Periods of Deload:

Your training strategy should include scheduled deload intervals to aid with recovery, avoid overtraining, and encourage long-term development.

During deload weeks or mesocycles, lower training volume and intensity for a brief period of time to allow for both psychological and physiological recovery while preserving training consistency.

Comments and Modifications:

To maximize training stimulation and growth, pay attention to the signals your body is giving you and modify sets and reps accordingly.

Be adaptable and prepared to modify your training regimen in light of trainee feedback, evolving conditions, and training objectives.

Through the implementation of progressive overload, periodization, tracking, and feedback systems in your sets and reps program, you may optimize strength, muscle growth, endurance, and performance while also managing training volume and intensity and promoting ongoing adaptation.

Summary

In conclusion, a variety of elements, such as your fitness goals, training experience, personal preferences, and unique needs, influence how many sets and repetitions you should perform. There is no one-size-fits-all method when it comes to sets and repetitions, regardless of your goals: increasing muscle mass, strength, endurance, or general fitness.

When creating your exercise regimen, it's critical to comprehend the concepts of progressive overload, periodization, and individualization. You may maximize your training results and make significant progress by gradually increasing training volume and intensity over time, adjusting sets and reps based on your experience level and goals, and customizing your program to fit your unique requirements and preferences.

Always pay attention to your body's signals, monitor your development, and modify your sets and repetitions in response to feedback and performance metrics. You may control training variables, promote adaptation, and ultimately meet your fitness objectives by using a methodical yet adaptable approach to sets and reps.

The number of sets and repetitions that you should perform vary from person to person, thus there is no hard and fast rule. Try out various set and rep schemes to see what suits you the best. In your fitness quest, never stop trying to get better.

THE END

www.ingramcontent.com/pod-product-compliance
Lightning Source LLC
Chambersburg PA
CBHW051920250726
48659CB00002B/753